Born in Glasgow in the 1960s, Kenny Boden soon realised that life would be easier if you possessed either fast legs or a quick wit. All that running sounded too exhausting. His humour has been honed on 'through life' experiences and has proven invaluable currency. In his long police career, it provided a safety net facilitating more "Talk Downs" than "Take Downs". In later life, he has written a number of successful comedy scripts and continues to perform on the after-dinner circuit.

Kevin Hanretty worked as a consultant obstetrician and gynaecologist in the NHS for over twenty-five years. He looked after women with complicated pregnancies including morbid obesity and those with twin and triplet pregnancies in a busy city hospital. He has also worked in South Africa and Qatar He is relearning trumpet, learning piano and still needs to lose a bit more weight.

To Anne and Mary, thank you for your continued patience!
With thanks to: Rachael, Sophie Andrews, Carol Watson,
Isobel Gaudoin, Stona Fitch, Sally Clarke and Liz Tait

Thank you Isobel!
Yours Aye
Kenny.

Ps-page 69's tribute!

Kevin Hanretty MD and
Kenny W Boden

HOW TO BE A FAT LOSER

AUSTIN MACAULEY PUBLISHERS™

LONDON • CAMBRIDGE • NEW YORK • SHARJAH

A CIP catalogue record for this title is available from the British Library.

ISBN 9781398480773 (Paperback)
ISBN 9781398480780 (ePub e-book)

www.austinmacauley.com

First Published 2023
Austin Macauley Publishers Ltd®
1 Canada Square
Canary Wharf
London
E14 5AA

The authors acknowledge that many conditions exist which can cause or contribute to obesity. A chapter which addresses some of the more common causes has been included in this book. We really do strongly advise anyone suffering from any of these conditions to keep in touch with their doctor or health practitioner to ensure continued awareness of up-to-date alternative treatment options and potential breakthroughs.

With that said, this book is aimed primarily at people like Kenny and Kevin who freely acknowledge Fork Control Failure but reckon they've plenty of company out there!

Why not join us as we share experiences, proffer advice and give tips on why we all should invest some time in 'having a right good look at ourselves' ...whilst we are still able.

Oh! And let's try to have some laughs along the way!

This Book Offers Calorie Free Food for Thought!

Introduction

A cop and a gynaecologist meet at a party. Although it sounds like the build up to a cheesy Seventies joke, the meeting brought together Kenny, a veteran policeman and Kevin, a consultant gynaecologist/obstetrician. Both worked in the West of Scotland and despite such different vocations, shared a similar (dark) sense of humour. Now a lot has been written about the black humour found among cops and medics. The reality is, however, much of this has been honed from daily exposure to life at the sharp end, and acts like a pressure release valve. This can be helpful in preventing ludicrously high stress levels or the sudden urge to punch annoying people quite hard in the face.

Both had written some stuff. Kevin had published several undergraduate medical books and had a number of medical papers to his name. Admittedly, they were more humerus than humorous, but Kenny, after participating in new comedy writers' workshops, had sold comedy sketches to the BBC.

At this time, after too much food and certainly too much alcohol, they discussed collaborating on a writing project.

It was to be some years later before the perfect subject matter manifested because, in the intervening years, Kenny, age 46, had a life-changing encounter. A routine GP check-up found he had high blood pressure (HBP), high cholesterol, Type 2 diabetes...and obesity (thrown in to make a big round number presumably!)

Whilst these diagnoses shouldn't have come as a surprise, the experience felt like an axe attack.

The reality was that Kenny was addicted to sugar, his diet, weight and general health were spiralling out of control and he knew something had to be done...at some point.

Kenny's initial remedial efforts were as wobbly as a Weight Watcher's dance class. After repeated false starts, bolstered by multifarious excuses, the reality of his situation finally registered. With frequent medication hikes amid increasingly grim-sounding health warnings by medical experts, the head in the sand time was up.

Obesity and Type two diabetes are a really ugly partnership, producing health consequences that would make a Hollywood horror writer flinch. Blindness, premature deaths and limb amputations occur with alarming frequency.

Kenny got really spooked when realising that the writing was literally on the wall for him (or his lower limbs), when spotting a poster advertising a diabetic clinic's information session about potential diabetes damage to the blood vessels in the feet.

'Feet – How Important Are They?'

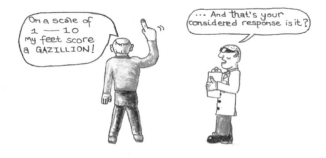

The actual wording on the poster

At this point Kenny drew on the wisdom of that age-old saying: "Fuck this, I need to do something now" and did something.

Right there. Right then.

A 47-pound weight drop and sub-25 Body Mass Index (BMI) score later, Kenny took back control of his lifestyle, and remains at a healthy weight to this day. On reflection, once the decision to act was reached, the journey was easier than expected. In fact, more of a lifestyle tweak than major overhaul.

Enter Kevin, and the intrepid duo forged an alliance to tackle obesity by bringing experience from both sides of the spectrum, namely the sufferer and a hospital consultant.

Indeed, on a daily basis, Kevin faced growing challenges. Obesity levels continue to climb, especially amongst pregnant women. Although mothers-to-be are expected to grow bigger naturally, being obese exacerbates any potential pregnancy concerns for both mother and baby. It can also lead to frustration amongst practitioners whose job just got much more complicated when it didn't have to. Of course, advising people of that fact often proves easier said than done.

No one (except perhaps sumo wrestlers) enjoy being told they're fat. That news can come as a shock to the system – akin to a stranger suddenly slapping your gran. Notwithstanding, such information IS crucial to the well-being of mother and child.

There is undoubtedly a balance to be struck. Firstly, some overweight patients may need to suck it up a bit and not feel obliged to have everything, including potentially lifesaving advice, sugar coated (pun fully intended!). As for doctors, some may have to realise that their bedside manner may not be as good as they think it is. In fact, many folks have encountered doctors who are to diplomacy what earthworms are to sandwiches.

Food for thought on both sides if anyone still has an appetite!

Oh! And another issue affecting Kevin, was his guilty secret. He himself had a higher than healthy BMI and when dispensing weight-related advice, felt like the crowned king of hypocrites!

Seeking to tackle a serious and literally growing problem in a more palatable fashion, they hope that their humour (even if a bit gruesome) serves as a veritable 'spoonful of sugar' (or sweetener!) to help digest the shockingly gungy bits.

The writers are acutely aware that writing about a deeply personal and sensitive topic such as obesity, without causing some offence, would be akin to navigating a minefield wearing a blindfold and clown shoes.

They foster a genuine belief however, that much like climate change, obesity has a pivotal point, when the road back to good health will seem insurmountable or in fact be closed. This book seeks not to 'Fat Shame', but rather to help readers 'Fat Tame'. The message is just way too important to ignore.

We do, however, caution readers of a delicate disposition, to either put the book down and walk away, or sit back and put on a sensitivity seatbelt – It could be a bumpy ride!

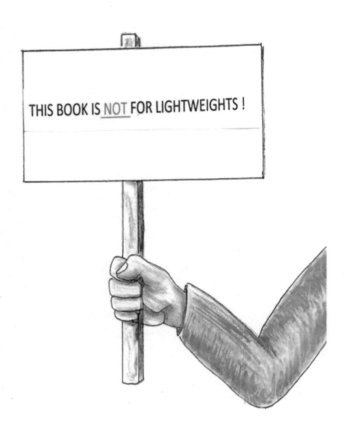

"Doc, I'm just big-boned, I'm not really fat
But you'll just have to take my word for that
I see by your face that you think I'm in denial
But this is a free country, and I'm not on trial.
As my GP you're supposed to lighten my load
So, get my name right, it's Mr Todd not Mr Toad!

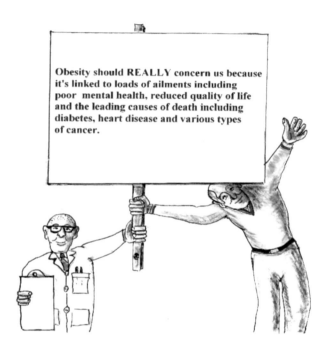

The Doc and Mr Don't Know

Why Do We Need
This Kind of Book?

Why do we need this kind of book? Because nobody seems to be listening! At least 2.8 million people die each year as a result of being overweight or obese.

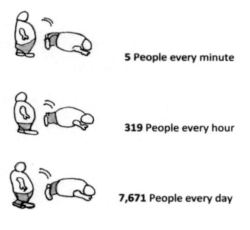

5 People every minute

319 People every hour

7,671 People every day

As early as 1997, the World Health Organisation recognised obesity as a worldwide problem. Then along comes another pandemic that 'Tag Teams' with obesity. The Covid-19, or Coronavirus outbreak, is killing and damaging people in almost every country in the world and is, understandably, being treated as a significant health risk.

What is particularly alarming is the connection between the two pandemics: The chances of being admitted to an intensive care unit with Covid (and other bad things) is four times greater for people with a high BMI compared to folk with normal weight.

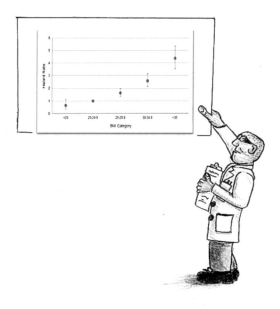

As BMI increases, all of the medical risks of Covid, for example admission to Intensive Care Units, increases dramatically.

As a species we're getting fatter, faster. Since 1975 obesity rates have almost tripled. Around 30% of the world's population is now overweight or obese – nearly two billion folks! More than half of the children in the US will become obese adults. In the UK the NHS budget is as stretched as a fat bloke's pants, with more and more resources being channelled into obesity-related ailments.

In 2018/2019 there were 876,000 UK hospital admissions where obesity was reported as a factor, up a massive 23% from the year before.

Whilst around 30,000 deaths every year in the UK are a result of obesity, this is way less than the number killed by Covid in 2020. The good news is that Covid will eventually be controlled if not eradicated by vaccination.

The bad news is that obesity won't. Vaccines can prevent susceptibility to coronavirus in the obese but can't prevent overeating.

Whilst loads of factors exist which can increase the likelihood of obesity, a lack of self-control remains a major contributor.

This is not a diet book. Rather, it attempts to provide a realistic, if possibly disturbing, take on the actual dangers of carrying excess weight, hoping to offer a viable case for a lifestyle change.

If global obesity levels were to be likened to a runaway train, this book seeks to convince readers why they really, really, should get off at the next available stop!

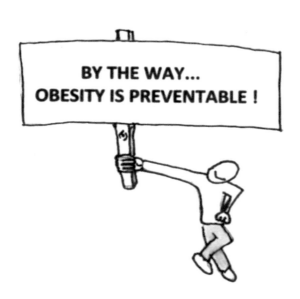

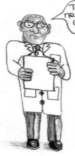
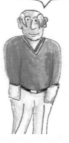

The Doc and Mr Don't Know

My doctor let out such a disdainful sigh
Whilst announcing the results of my BMI
He said it was the highest he'd ever seen
And for my weight I should be 8 feet 14.

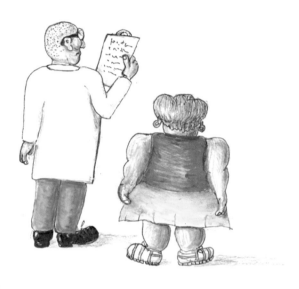

BMI or Body Mass Index is that much maligned measurement model, calculated by dividing our weight in kilograms by our height in metres squared. Most people have heard of it. But it's got lots of limitations and nobody seems to have a good word about it.

The idea is that just knowing we're 15 stone (95 kg) tells very little about how much fat we might be carrying. If you're 4 feet 9 inches and 15 stone, then your BMI is 45 which is way high – akin to poking the grim reaper with a stick! But if you're the same weight and 6 feet 4 inches your BMI is 25 and totally healthy.

If BMI is less than 18.5, we're deemed underweight and if our BMI is 18.5 to 25, we fall in the healthy range.

However, if our BMI is 25 to 30, we're overweight and if our BMI is 30 or higher, we're officially obese and sailing in dangerous waters, health-wise.

BMI is almost certainly not the most accurate way to gauge a healthy weight, but it does give us a general idea, a starter for ten if you will.

If we exercise regularly, eat sensibly and generally look after our body, we'd probably be right in suspecting a BMI of more than 25 didn't really reflect our true health risk but if we spend our day shuffling between cake shops, don't be surprised when our BMI is sky-high.

Something Has to Give

Let's look at things from a different angle.

Let's imagine that our weight is now measured in cans/tins of soup. We'll take it that a standard can weighs around 16 oz.

That means being two stone overweight would equate to roughly 28 cans and four stone overweight would equate to 52 cans. And so on.

"Mr Campbell...you're a 100 canner."

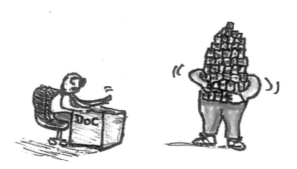

The point of this exercise is to choose a medium which lets us experience (if we wanted to) what our excess weight would feel like being physically carried. Arguably, a '14 canner' (@ one stone) could walk about for a while before the load became too heavy...or just really annoying.

However, many of us are ten stone or more above our recommended healthy weight. (That's a staggering 140 plus cans).

Rather incredibly, most of us would be unable to physically lift our 'can cargo'. And yet we choose to carry that weight 24/7, 365, as body fat.

But, at some point, whether it's the arse of our pants, our dignity or our health…something's got to give.

Damaged joints, HBP, and now diabetes
Is this really the way you want to treat us?
You've no control and eat what you like
Continue on, and I may go on strike
Stop pigging out or results may be shocking
Please listen to me. This is your body talking.

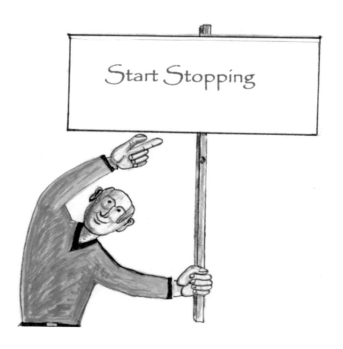

Start Stopping

Life can be cruel and, even with today's medical advances, navigating a healthy passage through to HEALTHY old age without attracting serious illness is found in only about 5 % of the population. That means nine out of ten of us may experience bad health. We then hear that an estimated six of the ten leading factors contributing to disease globally are lifestyle related.

And here's the thing…

There is a difference between life expectancy and Healthy Life Expectancy (HLE). In the period 2015 to 2017, men in the UK had a life expectancy of 79.2 years but their HLE was 63.1 years. Women had a life expectancy of a whopping 82.9 years but their HLE was only 63.6 years. Whilst the good news may be that we are all expected to live longer, the not so good news is that, partly due to the damage previously done to joints by carrying too much weight, that extra time can be fairly miserable and begin to feel like eternity!

Worryingly, this eating epidemic knows no boundaries or social barriers, crossing all continents, ages, sexes, and intellects. From tubby teachers, dumpy doctors and porky politicians to overweight oldies and chunky children, we are rapidly becoming a big fat world.

There is so much talk now about the 'new normal' but carrying too much weight has become the new normal for so many of us. We learn to live with it and our workaround is by buying bigger sizes without taking any notice until our health is affected.

If Darwin were alive today, he might just have to rethink his human evolution theory.

THE ASCENT OF MAN...
DESCENT

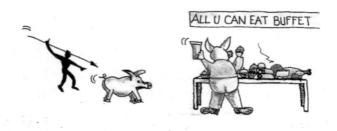

I eat when I'm hungry
I eat when I'm alone
Whilst watching telly
Or chatting on the phone

I eat when I get worried
And eat when I'm annoyed
When I'm down in the dumps
Or when my hopes are buoyed

I eat when I'm nervous
And also when I'm bored
When I come to think of it
Why's my weight soared?

I'll award myself a biscuit if I can solve this mystery!

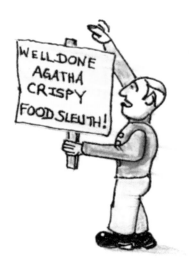

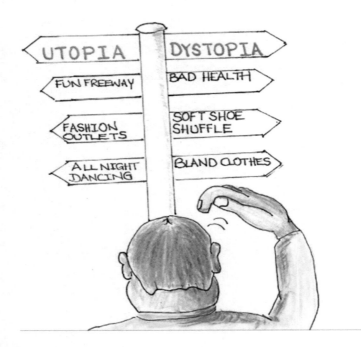

Utopia Versus Dystopia

We'll need to draw on our imagination to envisage the nature of this section because it may not have happened...yet!

In the perfect world, or utopia, we would all be healthy. Interestingly, according to the World Health Organisation very few of us would be, under their definition of health – in 'a state of complete physical, mental and social well-being and not merely the absence of disease or infirmity.'

In other words, even if we think being 'curvy' or 'big boned' isn't a problem, it certainly isn't a healthy place to be.

An imagined utopia, as in that perfect place to be, for folk with excess weight issues, would almost definitely include being a healthy weight and having a figure or physique that impressed us when we looked in a mirror. (We wouldn't have to hold our tummy in anymore!).

We would dress in clothing that now complemented our shape and attracted positive comment from others. Also, as a direct consequence of having our weight within our control, our general health would be better too. We could easily imagine a newfound confidence enabling all sorts of social and employment opportunities. And so, the list goes on...

Sound farfetched? It isn't – been there. Done that. Still doing it...and it's fabby!

An imagined dystopia, for folk with weight issues, really could be a nightmare. As more weight goes on, interest or indeed ability to participate in physical activity, including sex, dwindles. Clothing choice becomes what fits, rather than what favours. Bad health beckons and with it a growing dependency on medication and treatments.

Less and less control of our own life follows, and with it, dramatically reduced lifestyle options.

Sounds farfetched? It's not – ask any of the 700 million obese folks on the planet if that description rings any bells.

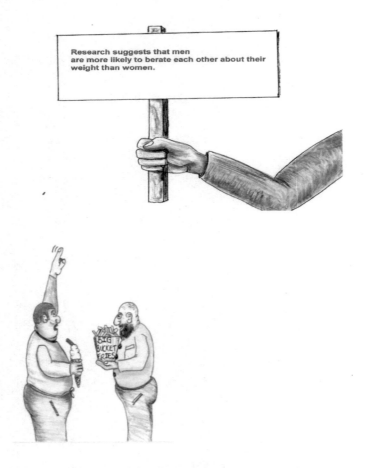

Research suggests that men are more likely to berate each other about their weight than women.

'Don't believe everything you read, tubster.'

Benefits of Non-Obesity...

A reduced chance of contracting major illnesses – even modest weight loss reduces blood pressure and improves blood sugar levels. Arguably the most important benefit is increased self-esteem – almost all studies looking at self-esteem showed improvements following weight reduction interventions.

The health benefits of weight loss are numerous.

Just some of them can be shown here:

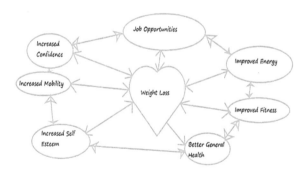

The key point here is that weight loss leads to increased energy which leads to improved fitness which leads to better health etc, etc...but all of this feedback to aid further weight loss which in turn leads to improved self-esteem etc. etc.

For some of us, this needs signposted.

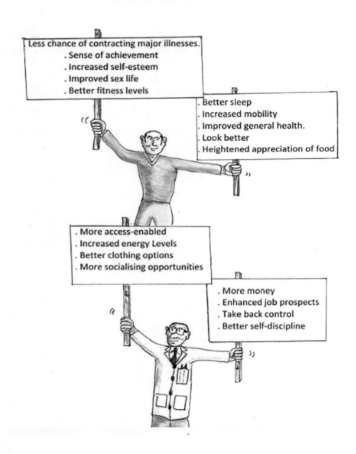

BENEFITS OF NON-OBESITY

Less chance of contracting major illnesses.
. Sense of achievement
. Increased self-esteem
. Improved sex life
. Better fitness levels

. Better sleep
. Increased mobility
. Improved general health.
. Look better
. Heightened appreciation of food

. More access-enabled
. Increased energy Levels
. Better clothing options
. More socialising opportunities

. More money
. Enhanced job prospects
. Take back control
. Better self-discipline

Benefits of Being Obese –

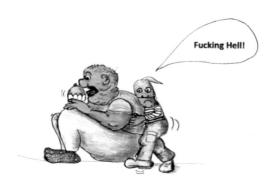

Less likely to be stolen!

We all know that the path to healthy longevity is not guaranteed and whilst crossing our fingers and hoping for the best is unlikely to change much, living it 'too large' just might. Carrying excess weight doesn't guarantee illness but it can massively increase the odds of bringing it to your door. It's a bit like strapping a raw steak to our body and jumping into a shark tank…

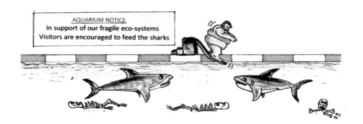

Talking About Obesity Should Not Be A 'Blame Game'

As we've said before, various factors such as medical and socio-economic conditions exist, causing or worsening weight gain but for a vast number of us, we really do have to accept some responsibility for our own actions.

Blaming the government, food manufacturers or sugar producers for our body shape is like taking umbrage at images of cream cakes for being too damn attractive! Surely if we know that eating too much is potentially harmful, but continue stuffing our faces anyway, that's down to us.

On the face of it, it seems that without portion police monitoring our fork control or calorie courts sentencing us to salad camp, many of us just have to accept that we are pretty shit at self-discipline.

In fact, it's almost as if we worship some strange deity who chips away at our resolve every waking moment...

Aw-Fuck-It

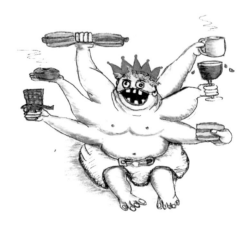

God of Sweet Temptations

Meet Aw-Fuck-It, God of Sweet Temptations and Master of Influence. This forceful mind entity is the go-to guy when we need a readymade excuse or an 'out' from common sense. A constant presence that can always be relied upon to say what we want to hear!

Don't think you're familiar with his work? See if anything registers amongst the following phrases – usually uttered by us when dangling some calorie-ridden monster morsel or delish drink inches from our face!

'Aw-Fuck-It…you only live once… So live it large'
(Bariatric funerals are now available)

'Aw-Fuck-It…diets don't work anyway'
(Ever stop and wondered why?)

'Aw-Fuck-It… Something's got to kill you'
(With many additional variants for obese folks!)

'Aw-Fuck-It… I'm on holiday/it's the weekend'
(NB our digestive systems need breaks too!)

Damn That Kitchen

We all know the story. We set out full of good intentions, planning to have a day of responsible eating. And the plan works, right up to the second we walk into our kitchen. We have just entered the cravings capital of the world and domain of AW-FUCK-IT, god of sweet temptation. Tasty morsels lie everywhere, calling our name. Whilst the urge to feast is enormous, there are a few tried and tested pointers to help resist:

Drink Water on Entry – When entering the kitchen, get into the habit of making straight for the tap and drinking a glass of water. At times hunger pangs are confused with thirst.

Eye Level Is Buy Level – This is the mantra of retailers who know that items placed at eye level sell better. The idea then, is to NEVER have snacks lying about in sight within the kitchen, thus reducing the likelihood of snacking whilst preparing food.

Be Realistic – When counting calories – very, very few of us accurately count the calorie values of food. There is a tendency to ignore dressings, nibbles, salad and fruit items. If we got better at it, it would make a big difference in the amounts we actually ate, and the weight we subsequently lost. Keeping a notepad in the kitchen and noting down EVERYTHING we eat can be enlightening…or downright frightening!

The Right Plate Size

Many factors prevent maintenance dieting and one common one, believe it or not is plate size. There is some controversy about this, but the use of bigger plates is followed by the temptation to cover the plate with food which in turn drives the urge to finish that food accompanied by a desire not to waste it.

Using the Kitchen

In truth a lot of us mostly use the kitchen to store cutlery needed for our Chinese, Indian or Italian carry-outs. So, while carry-outs are fabby and a great treat, we should try to have them as an occasional treat. Because fast food is a bona fide way to fast weight gain.

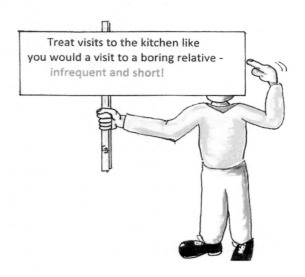

Treat visits to the kitchen like you would a visit to a boring relative - infrequent and short!

Getting Real

A magical wee story...

Imagine you are walking through an enchanted forest when you meet a kindly wizard.

The wizard assures you he can make you feel much better with one of his 'Happy Spells'.

Using his magic, the wizard alters your shape, transforming you into a slimmer version of yourself.

On seeing the new you emerge, you instantly feel better, loving the new look.

The wizard then tells you that there's more good stuff to come, as the spell will also give you a better chance of good health, and more money to spend. The wizard tells you that this is to help you live happily ever after.

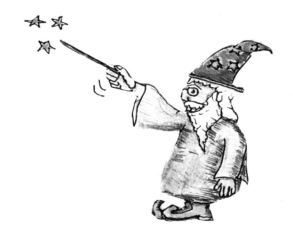

Get real Gandalf – 'enchanted forest' stories are for kids.

PS. The wizard in the story is actually YOU – so go work your own magic!

Who Can Help?

Whilst being obese definitely makes us far more likely to visit a doctor in respect of the multifarious ailments caused or exacerbated by too much fat, just how well would doctors actually perform as an overweight patient's first point of contact when seeking help to lose weight?

Clearly, we want to avoid stereotypes and generalisations but, as outlined in our introduction, not all doctors are particularly good at dealing with obesity. Maybe part of that is down to what they think when they see us. As we know, doctors study and train hard and, as a global body, can tackle most known and emerging medical conditions. They pride themselves on that and, like most professionals, are 'in it to win it'. They want to succeed and are up for the challenge, but perhaps can feel a bit frustrated that we've tipped the scales against that (pun fully intended!).

All doctors sign up to a duty of care in respect to patients which, put simply, means they undertake to always have our best health interests at heart. But surely, we too have a duty of care…to ourselves?

It's like the old joke where, believing they're down on their luck, a person repeatedly prays to their god, extolling their own virtues and demanding intervention to help win the state lottery. Eventually their god replies, asking, "Can you at least try to meet me halfway…by buying a lottery ticket?"

It begs the question of why wouldn't we at least try to help our doctor help us? Any weight loss process will work so much better if it can be a reciprocal arrangement. And in so doing we answer the chapter heading question of 'Who can help me?'

And, by the way, no one escapes that advice:

I like chocolate, pies and peas
Trifle, shortbread, cakes and cheese
Sandwiches, sausages, ice cream and jelly
Everything possible I can stuff in my belly

I graze all day, sleep, reload
I'm now concerned I may explode
I must cut down on the food I sample
As a doctor I'm setting a bad example.

Exercise should be a balance between what we want to do and what we can do. Running suits some people. Doing weights in the gym suits others.

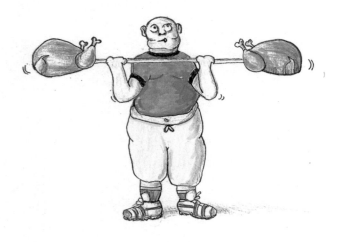

Remember, other forms of exercise can be effective too.

Nude Street Dancing

Get naked, take to the streets, crank up the music and really shake them floppy bits! With all that frenetic movement, the calories will soon burn off.

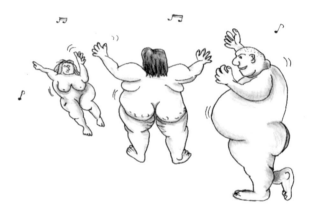

Particularly when the police arrive!

The Other Side of the Scale

We're all guilty of it. Scouring the labels of tasty foodstuffs, trying to work out if scoffing it down would overwhelm our recommended daily amount of calories. *

What happens though if we do go over our healthy parameters, feel guilty, and feel the need to burn off those extra calories? Current food labelling doesn't provide information on the amount or type of exercise required to burn off calories.

Recent research however suggests that trials with labelling which did so, helped people make a more informed choice, and as a direct consequence, led to a reduction in calorie intake.

*Guideline Daily Amount equals 2500 cals for a man, 2000 cals for a woman.

Obviously, exercising DOES burn calories but results depend on a whole bag of variables, from our weight to exercise type, the speed at which the exercise is conducted, and so on. So, with that in mind, the following example should be regarded as a 'rough' guide to how many calories we may lose by walking.

We'll base our table on a person weighing 180 pounds, with the rule of thumb estimate of 100 calories being burnt off by every mile walked.

Now, let's look at this information from a different perspective. What, if instead of trying to shed the calories through exercise after the event, we had to walk the equivalent distance to reach the food in the first place? Boy oh boy, would that make a difference to our choices…and our shapes!

ITEM	CALORIES	DISTANCE
Chocolate Biscuit	200	2 miles
Pizza	1800	18 miles
Kebab	2000	20 miles
All You Can Eat Buffet	5000	50 miles

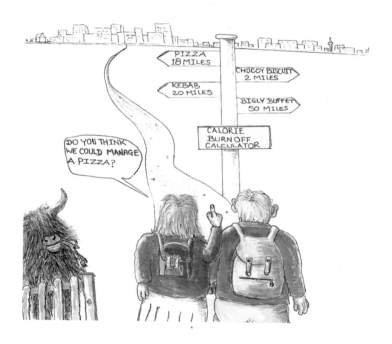

Top Tip

Seven Deadly Sins: Envy, Greed, Sloth, Lust, Gluttony, Pride and Wrath.

If you feel the need to participate in any of the seven deadly sins, we suggest lust over gluttony, greed or sloth…as there's a chance of burning off more calories!

Human beings can be incredibly bad at evaluating risk. A recent example is people exiting shops and taking off their face masks in order to light up a cigarette. In reality their chance of dying of Covid is a fraction of the chance of dying from smoking related disease. It is the urgency of the threat that prompts action.

For some people this might whilst attending an infertility clinic to be told that only with considerable weight loss are they likely to achieve a pregnancy. Sadly, with regard to things like pregnancy, perceived as a happy, joyful and natural time, the complications are increasing dramatically due to a more than doubling of the proportion of obese pregnant women in the last 20 years.

For others it may be in finding out their worn and painful hip joints won't be replaced until they too have achieved significant weight loss.

We often disregard risks until they are forced upon us but, if you ever felt the need to unblock your bowels, disrupt your sleep pattern or experience more anxiety than cramped cattle on an abattoir road trip, imagine yourself standing face to face with a consultant oncologist (cancer specialist) waiting to hear your test results. (I think we'd probably all agree that any health worker onerously tasked with delivering potentially life changing news, tops the list of people most capable of frightening the living bejeezus out of us!)

Interestingly, during such consultations, which occur everywhere, every day, many people decide (regardless of whether the news is good or not), to quit their excesses. There and then, a decision to stop drinking, smoking or overeating is made because that long term habit suddenly became far less important.

The point is that we CAN actually stop unhealthy behaviour just as soon as we want to, when we feel we need to. So, in order to avoid any of the above scenarios becoming real, probably best not to wait for that short, sharp, shock!

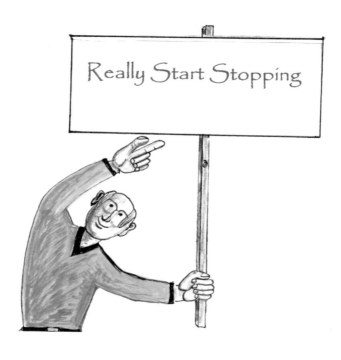

'Suffer the Little Children'

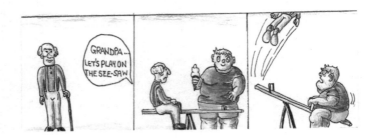

- Children are more likely to be overweight or obese if their parents are.
- Figures suggest children with two obese parents can be 10 to 12 times more likely to be obese.
- Overweight and obese children are more likely to stay obese into adulthood.
- Childhood obesity is associated with a higher likelihood of premature death and disability in adulthood.

We're just saying...

The Doc and Mr Don't Know

Question: I'm a 37-year-old man carrying a bit of weight around my waist. Could this be puppy fat?

Mr Don't Know:
Not unless you own a fat puppy
And you're holding it at your waist.

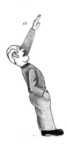

Doc: The term 'puppy fat' refers to fat on the body of a baby or child which disappears around adolescence.

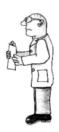

Hormones

If I speak to my daughter about her weight
we both end up getting into a bit of a state
for me to comment sounds quite pathetic
I'm also overweight... And fear it's genetic.

Hormones and Other (Mostly) Myths

"I think he's just big boned, doctor." Or "It's just her hormones, doctor." These are frequent comments from parents about their overweight children. But is that the case?

Of course, there are conditions that are associated with being overweight. The classic one is of an underactive thyroid gland which can affect both men and women. The thyroid controls metabolic rate and if it is not working properly can slow it up, then we simply cannot use the calories we take in. So, we put on weight, become really constipated and our hair and skin suffer.

In women, periods can also become chaotic and heavy.

The good news is that treatment for an underactive thyroid is usually straightforward, using tablets to replace the thyroid hormone that's lacking.

Other less common hormone problems affect the adrenal glands which control many things like salt and fluid balance, blood pressure and urine production and are also implicated in weight gain.

By far the greatest culprit amongst women is Polycystic Ovary Syndrome which probably affects up to 10% of women. It is associated with weight gain, oily skin, facial hair and, rather tragically, infertility. The cause remains unknown.

Many people blame being overweight on PCOS but given that there are lots more people who are known to be overweight than actually have PCOS, this looks like another example of blame game.

Here's the Important Bit

Whilst the role of PCOS in making people overweight may not be fully understood yet, what is known is that the best treatment is not hormones or complicated operations... It's weight loss.

The same goes for overweight people who may have fertility issues. Losing weight improves the prospects for successful treatment enormously.

So, for most of us, if it's not hormones, not being big boned or 'genetic', then why are we overweight?

Whilst we now know that many factors exist which can increase the likelihood of obesity, a lack of self-control remains a major contributor.

Many of us may buy diet books or recipe books in the hope that they might help self-control... They probably won't.

This is not a diet book. Rather, it attempts to provide a realistic, if possibly disturbing, take on the actual dangers of carrying excess weight, hoping to offer a viable case for a lifestyle change.

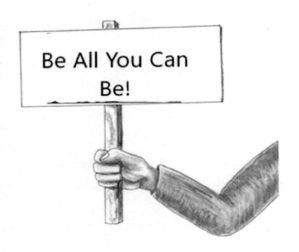

Self Scunner Technique

We've all been there. We plonk down on the sofa to eat our TV dinner just as a nature programme shows a scene of a mass of writhing maggots within a dead carcass. Suddenly our chicken fried rice loses its appeal as our appetite is temporarily shut down.

What you may not know is that this 'scunner-switch' is actually practised by some whilst trying to shed or maintain their existing weight. This is done using the mental imagery of gross scenes to stave off unwanted hunger pangs, particularly in respect of hedonistic hunger.

(Scunner: Scottish word for 'a strong dislike.')

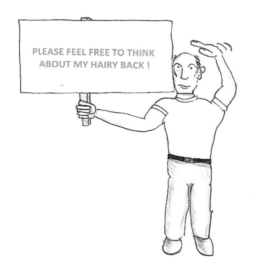

Even if that idea keeps away the hunger pangs—always remember!

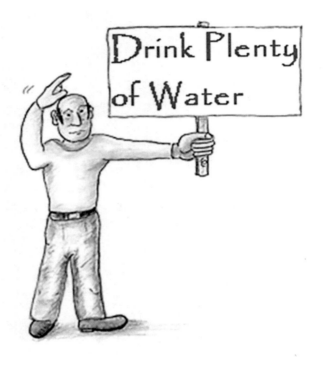

Not only can drinking water help reduce hunger pangs, it can flush out crap like a plumber on overtime!

Our Beautiful Big Brain and How to Use It

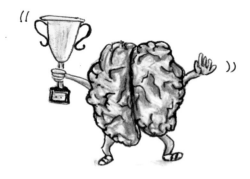

Our brains are just amazing. The best of the best. Bigly capable.

Nothing in the known universe exists which is truly comparable. A super-duper, supercomputer if you will. Artificial intelligence may be the latest would-be usurper, but for it to fully supplant the brain, we will have to wait a while! Whilst the brain's full capabilities still remain uncharted, here are but a tiny fraction of good bits: It's **a time machine** – able to instantly transport us back to a distant memory, in colour, with sound.

We can be back in conversations with late loved ones or checking out our bloody awful fashion choices of yesteryear.

It's a giant **vault of knowledge** – facts and figures instantaneously brought to mind – without having to wait about for a bored librarian with a wobbly trolley to bring our stuff.

Imagination – Einstein himself said *imagination is more important than knowledge.* Most human progress is due to mankind's imagination.

Just ask children to describe what a monster looks like and sit back. The variation in results will be amazing.

Incredible Skill Set –

Body repair shop – Free medical checks and treatment 24/7 – our brain constantly directs the equivalent of a gazillion mini doctors and nurses scuttling around inside us, checking our vital signs and fixing stuff where they can. Our brain can even repair itself!

Learning while we sleep – it's not uncommon for people to try in vain to learn a new skill, only to wake up from a sleep or dream on the desired task and realise they now have the skill.

Cognitive rehearsal – the ability to imagine a future scenario and see yourself dealing with the challenges of that situation. This is used by emergency personnel attending serious accidents to prepare for often grisly scenes.

Predictiveness

We can think of one word and, instantly, associated words in our mind flag up, usually in the order of ones we use most often. Where do you think the predictive texting concept originated? Try it with an expression like "He was renowned for having a massive…" (Really? A body part was the first thing that sprang to mind? Honestly!)

But the best thing about our brain is we all get one at birth, it's completely unique and we own it outright from the word go. Nothing we could ever own, ever, could be more valuable to us. If the truth were told however the brain's full capabilities remain beyond most of our comprehensions. And, as a result many of us are probably a bit guilty of underestimating how intelligent we are… Or could be (Yeah, we know that there are exceptions. The scientific name for them is smart arses).

Despite genuinely possessing god-like powers and capabilities, many of us struggle to grasp the rudimentary concept of using our brain to help us shift some weight! That's a bit like owning a top of the range Rolls Royce but deciding to ride about on a decrepit old bike dragged from a canal instead.

It's probably true to say that, in many cases, given the choice, our brains would probably opt to bugger off from us, it's sad-sack host, and relocate somewhere its abilities were more appreciated. Say, perhaps becoming a careers' adviser for politicians.

"Call me if you ever want to learn anything... Anything at all!"

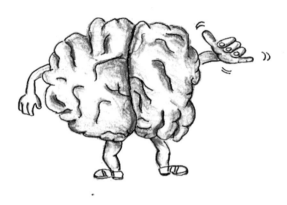

Over and above underusing our brains, comes another threat in the battle against obesity, in the form of HEDONIC HUNGER. This is described as the drive to eat to obtain pleasure in the absence of an energy deficit. In other words, we can develop cravings which make us eat simply because we want to and not because we have to. These cravings are similar to those which cause some people to gamble compulsively or use drugs recreationally. It is also similar to sexual cravings. And we all know what can happen when a person gets horny with nowhere to go with it!

Some of the ways to reduce hedonic hunger cravings are to remove food temptations from view or close proximity i.e., don't walk about with your pockets crammed with enough chocolate treats to open a Ferrero Rocher store.

"Right, that's me away to the shops..."

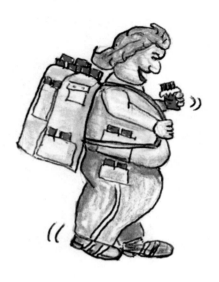

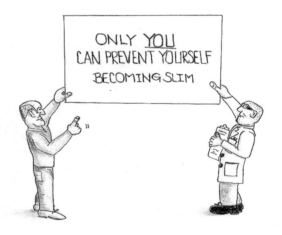

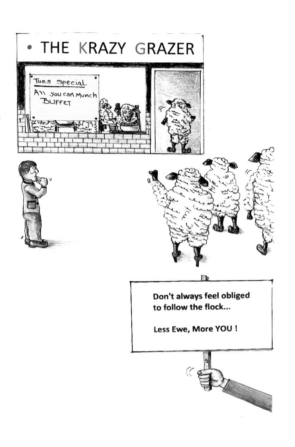

My slim pals drive me nutty
Their lives seem such a riot
Mine's the polar opposite
I'm ALWAYS on a diet
They seem to eat relentlessly
But no meat goes on the bone
I only have to read one recipe
And I put on half a stone.

Life in the Fast Lane

Wow! Is society changing... Or what?

Nowadays, we seem to want everything quick and easy. Everywhere, constantly, fingers are tapping furiously on tiny buttons, doing stuff. Whether channel surfing on TV, chewing the fat on social media or ordering superfluous junk from the internet, we want it just as fast as our podgy hands can press for it.

And more and more is being done from the comfort of our 'Sofa-Hub'. Mainstream sofas now come bigger than ever, loaded with more gizmos than a premium cinema seat; reclining cushions, footrests, food storage areas, cup holders, electric points and USB ports. At this rate they'll soon come with built-in toilets. Then, other than our bowels, we won't have to move much at all. (They'll probably name it the 'sit and shit' sofa).

"This new crappa-couch is fabby... Parp! We can now watch two full box sets without getting up... Parp!"

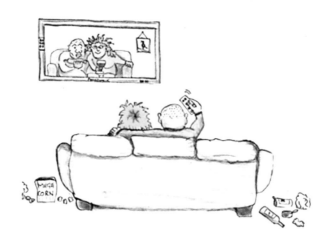

Somewhat ironically however, in the race to fill our lives with gadgets and services that are labour-saving, we seem to be losing interest in participating in any physical exertion with similar speed. This can lead to a vicious circle which sees us put on weight, become less inclined to exercise, which in turn, causes more weight gain. And so on.

The best thing to do to prevent the rut you're getting into becoming a trough, is to raise your respect for yourself, and for the tradition of eating itself.

Slouching in the sofa whilst grazing on food not only looks slobbish, it's pretty unhealthy too. We've got to make eating a little more special, more of an occasion if you will. Why not start having at least one meal a day at the table, where phones and the like are a no-no.

Then, simply take more time to enjoy the food and the banter!

The Doc and Mr Don't Know

Question: When's too heavy?

Mr Don't Know: Mmm. Perhaps this example will help. When buying a new vehicle, your priority is less the make, model or even colour. It's whether you can fit in it.

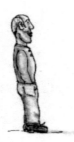

Doc: Wow! Actually, I'd probably start by establishing what my BMI was...

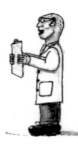

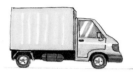

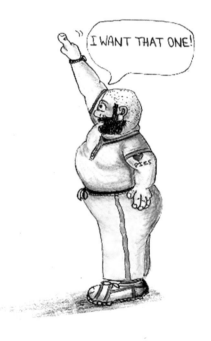

My tummy's so fat I can't see my feet
Belly button, penis or small folk I meet
My stomach has gotten so awfully round
It's 12 years since I've seen the ground
Walking has now become a real kerfuffle
Sideways waddling in the soft-shoe shuffle.

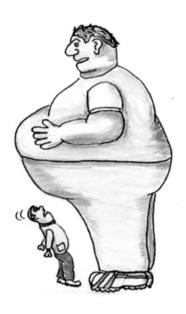

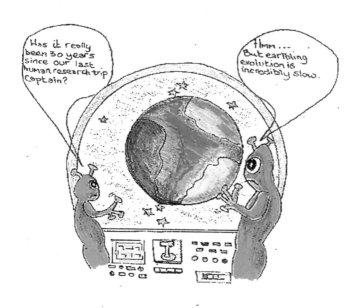

Earthbound Alien Abduction Craft

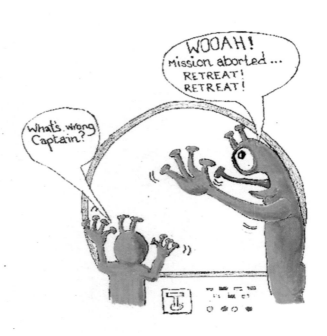

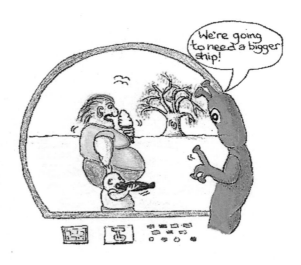

Diets are SO, SO boring
Like watching drying paint
Minutes and hours climb in my ear
Nibbling at my restraint.
Next, excuses flood my brain
My resolve is soon reduced
Four biscuits, three cakes later
And this diet just got goosed.

Diets and Us

The actual ability to successfully lose weight and keep it off, hinges on just one thing.

We Must Want to Do It.

The decision to want to do it is a balance between the comforts we may feel from eating and the consequences of being obese. If your personal balance is that you feel better eating than addressing the problems of obesity though, it may be that your scales are not the only things off balance.

Nobody, as in no one at all, can do it for us. Not friends, doctors, medicine, personal trainers, or health gurus.

Being honest about our excesses can feel liberating and is definitely a step in the right direction. It does, however, suggest a food imbalance, best described by the adage 'Intake needs to be less than output' when referring to food scoffed and calories burnt off through exercise. This sounds like the clichéd bit where everybody conjures up images that are unpleasant or boring or futile. But it can be done, and really isn't that difficult. It just needs to be approached from a different mindset.

What if we **never** really had to go on a diet again, ever? We just have to tweak our existing lifestyles a wee bit. The main stimulus for making the commitment lies in the answer to a simple question:

Q: Is it better being slimmer?

A: Abso-fucking-lutely!

Here's a bold statement – **Diets very seldom work in the long term.**

That's simply because they're unrealistic and demand abstinence from food we crave. Anyone who thinks 'That's so wrong! I've been on lots of successful diets', may just be missing the point.

Dieting requires the very same discipline that we lacked in the first place which, in turn, caused the need to go on the frigging diet!

So, let's be naughty for a moment and admit a few wee home truths:

Most of us like eating…and/or drinking.

Most of us will eat/drink if, and when, we want to.

Most of us like eating/drinking more than we like exercise.

Sometimes We Need to Make Difficult Decisions

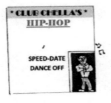

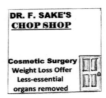

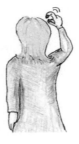

The Doc and Mr Don't Know

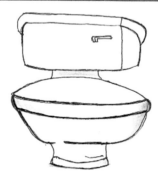

" Do you think the NHS will start naming their ever-increasing toilets like available coffee sizes? - This one could be the Crap-Achino Grande "

" Hopefully not "

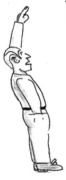

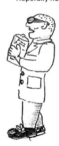

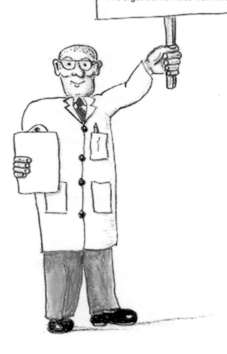

Kenny, at what point did you realise you were carrying an excessive amount of weight?

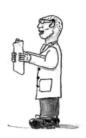

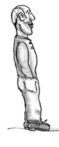

On reflection, the first clue should have been my direct debit with the local kebab shop. Actually it was when I realised my clothing size had more Xs than a Valentine's card from a randy lover.

The Doc and Mr Don't Know

Little White Lies...

And why the truth matters.

My friends all tell me porky pies
When making reference to my size
Their good intentions to protect
Serve to undermine my intellect

Yet I'm complicit in their little game
I've more insecurities than I can name
Their words do bring temporary peace
Masking the truth that I am obese

But imagine how good I'll really feel
When, with effort, I'm slim for real.

Humans are a social species and most of us like to be liked. There are of course exceptions to every rule. But let's leave the A-holes out of this for the moment!

If there really was a magic word in this life, it surely would – be BALANCE.

All things benefit from it – The solar system, nature, decisions, behaviour and eating!

What we must be aware of however, is our tendency to replace honesty with niceness. (We know, a 'can of worms' subject, but too important to ignore).

Let's look at potential answers to an often-asked question, and imagine it's asked by an overweight friend:

Question: Does my bum look big in this?

Possible responses:

Answer A: (Way Wrong:)

Fuck yeah! – You look like the victim of a madman run amok with an air compressor.

Answer B: (Just Wrong:)

Now I'm not saying you're fat – just a long way from slim.

Answer C: (Best yet but…)

Well, it's not particularly slimming, there are probably other things that would better suit your shape.

What we take from this scenario is that, if we feel obliged to ask that question of our friends or relatives, we probably already know the answer.

Ultimately, we're putting those close to us on the spot, hoping to allay our weight concerns or have our ego stroked. It may be time to accept that we are overweight, recognise it's not a crime and that we are certainly not alone.

Equally though, we should recognise that there's a straightforward way to feel better and attract genuine comments. We only live once but have control of how we want to be remembered.

Start valuing and investing in yourself more!

The Doc and Mr Don't Know

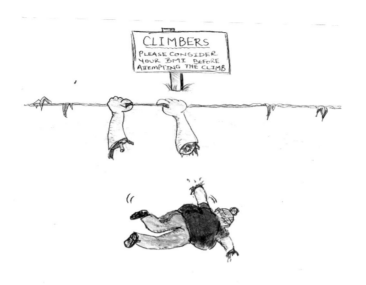

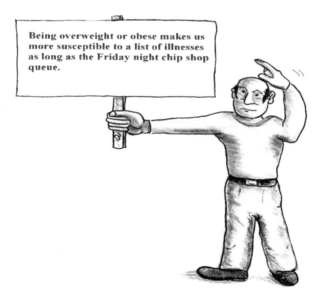

Being overweight or obese makes us more susceptible to a list of illnesses as long as the Friday night chip shop queue.

I like my food and enjoy having a bevvy
I also love fashion despite being heavy
Wearing haute couture, I exude style with sass
Unfortunately, my outfits often rip at the ass

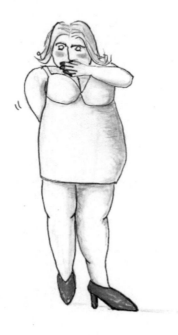

Shapewear

I'm not really as slim as folks think I am
The body form you see is a bit of a scam
My shape is a facade, a veritable veneer
But I can't do this without help, to be clear

My tummy control pants I squeeze on first
Using the strongest type in case they burst
Designed to be tight, fitting them can be hell
But hey! They're worth the effort as no VPL

Minimiser bra, followed by figure-hugging top
I can't really breathe but don't want to stop
Then on goes my face and my six-inch heels
Walking's murder. Can't stilettos have wheels?

Then went to a party and got asked to dance
I wanted to say yes but opted for 'no chance'
I was too worried that my outfit would give
You're probably thinking it's no way to live

As I've shown I can be determined and thrawn
Six months of restraint, my fat suit could be gone
I can lose weight. Of that there's no danger
I'll just focus on that dance with the stranger.

World's Best Investment

All we hear these days is investing, investing, investing. Making decisions on where to put our hard-earned cash. The choices are vast-stocks and shares, government bonds, rental properties, gold bars, alternative currency, solar energy or our dodgy mate Dougie's latest 'can't possibly fail' get-rich-quick scheme.

All of it, of course, is speculative where we hope to see our investment growing in value and, in the long term, turning into a nice little earner.

In other words, we're gambling with the chances of our investment's success.

Here's a sombre thought. Even if we did invest for the future really really wisely and all our investments came up smelling of roses. No cash, jewellery, luxury spas, sports cars, hair transplants or boob jobs are worth diddly-squat if we are dead or too ill to enjoy them.

We all saw how fragile our NHS was when swamped with demand for its resources during the first phases of the Covid-19 pandemic, and how grateful we were to its personnel for helping pull us through. The BBC has recently published an account of the impact Covid-19 had on NHS treatments: Around 4.7 million people were waiting for routine operations and procedures in England. The highest since 2007.

Nearly 380,000 people were waiting more than a year for non-urgent surgery compared with just 1600 before the pandemic began.

We have to reiterate that obesity is a bona fide growing global pandemic which no vaccine can cure.

Nor is there any cure-all operation or super drug which will work as a long-term investment – without us helping that process.

And this is where we make a prediction. The facts are clear that the NHS budget is under unprecedented pressure and changes will need to be made. The NHS is already making it MANDATORY that certain patients must lose weight before surgery, due to the risk of complications. We don't have to be an investment guru like Warren Buffett (pun intended) to predict many more such constraints being placed in the service and, possibly, not too distant future.

We can only hope that the NHS remains in better shape than many of us currently are.

So, what investment can bring us the best evidence of all? Investing in ourselves of course. Reaping the benefits of weight loss is off the scale fabulous!

We can start by enjoying special occasions, in terms of food/drink overload, even more, by making them just that- special and occasional. A bit like why Christmas is special – it's not every day. That would become samey monotonous very quickly. Anyway, who want to wash all those dishes?

So, whether we now decide to let the good times roll once a week, every weekend, or indeed just a step back from constantly grazing, why not do it? The best approach is probably the same as removing a sticking plaster i.e., don't faff about the edges – just get it done! Do it instantaneously, as in today not tomorrow or next week or when we can be arsed. We have to ask ourselves what 'planning' is really necessary when all we need do is put a bit less in our mouth each time we eat or drink? Start now... For your own sake. And if nothing else please consider this:

Money can't extend our life... But good health just might.

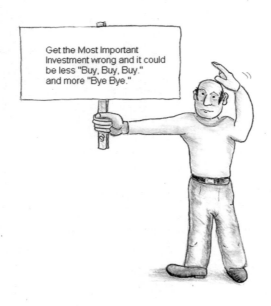

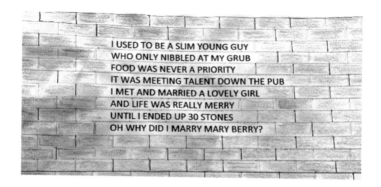

I USED TO BE A SLIM YOUNG GUY
WHO ONLY NIBBLED AT MY GRUB
FOOD WAS NEVER A PRIORITY
IT WAS MEETING TALENT DOWN THE PUB
I MET AND MARRIED A LOVELY GIRL
AND LIFE WAS REALLY MERRY
UNTIL I ENDED UP 30 STONES
OH WHY DID I MARRY MARY BERRY?

Imagine our body as a factory. If we tend to graze on food throughout our waking hours, our body will have to be working almost constantly to process all that food. As a factory owner, sooner or later we're likely to pay a price for exploiting our workforce.

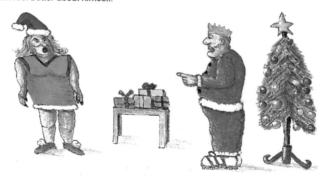

I've heard a rumour that Santa brings us loads of sweets at Christmas so we end up chubby like him, and he can feel better about himself.

What a load of rubbish! Who told you that? He actually does it so that we need to buy his oversized red onesies.

89

This Christmas I completely over-ate
And consumed it all at a glutton's rate
Now come January I must face the rap
That I've eaten gargantuan piles of crap

To make amends I've joined a gym
With the latest equipment to get me trim
My problem is the time I'm spending
On machines that are chocolate-vending!

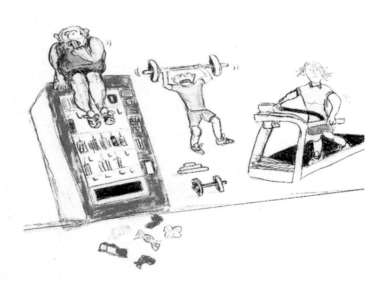

The Doc and Mr Don't Know

Question: Comments about my weight from colleagues at work hurt my feelings. What can I do about it?

Mr Don't Know: While stamping on their toes immediately springs to mind, revenge is best served cold. Get into shape, then get into their space and thank them. They will have no option but to capitulate!

Doc: That's actually a fair point. Channel negative comments into positive action. In other words, let the experience trigger your resolve.

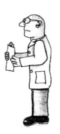

Shape Hiding

Well-chosen clothes can be slimming
but ultimately they can't tell lies
you'd have to dress in camouflage
to create that perfect disguise.

The Doc and Mr Don't Know

Question: I'm worried by   middle-aged creep.
What can I do?

Mr Don't Know:

I'd report it to
management at
work…or the
police.

Doc: Actually,
middle-aged
creep is Hard-
To-Shift weight
which can be
caused by
comfort eating
caused by stress.

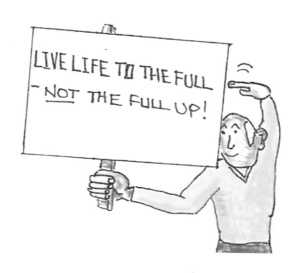

The Doc and Mr Don't Know

Question: I'd like to be a sugar daddy but I'm worried I'll get diabetes!

Mr Don't Know: Brilliant. I wish I'd thought of that line.

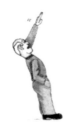

Doc: We can only hope he's kidding.

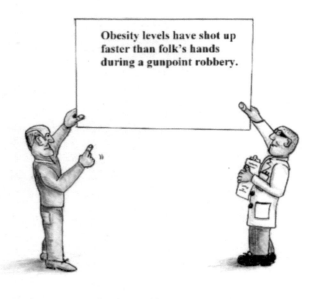

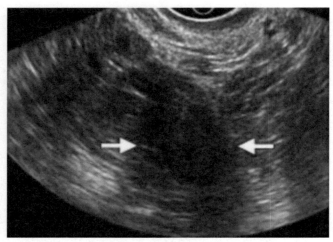

If you are overweight an Ultrasound scan can struggle to locate your baby or identify a significant number of problems which are also associated with obesity.

There is a baby in there but we just can't see it!

When I was heavy, no one referred to me as fatty
I don't remember any comments particularly catty
but getting into shape, after a calorie shedding spree
I attracted loads of comments complementary to me!

Get Wise to
your size.

The Doc and Mr Don't Know

Question: I hate drinking water. It's tasteless and disgusting. Can't I just take soft drinks?

Mr Don't Know:

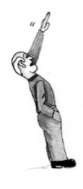
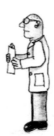

That reasoning would be the same as refusing surgery because you don't like the surgeon's shoes.

Doc: Water is incredible. It contains no calories but offers heaps of benefits including helping weight loss, increasing energy and improving skin to name a few. It has few competitors. Try squeezing in a lemon.

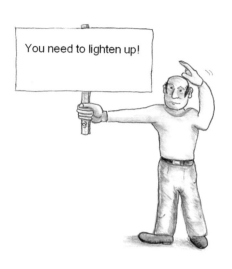

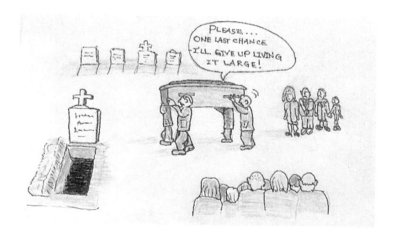

Funerals for the overweight are becoming more prevalent
and will almost certainly cost more, with morbidly obese
bodies weighing up to 600 pounds. To put that in perspective,
that's about the average weight of a piano. It is perhaps

somewhat understandable that funeral directors will seek to pass on investment costs. Funeral prices are likely to go up when factoring in the outlay for larger incinerators which are capable of accommodating larger bodies and the extra time required for burning the excess body fat. Additional costs can be added in the provision of bigger hearses and coffins and of course the heavy lifting gear necessary to move the coffin. The one thing we may end up getting a reduction on is dignity:

Here lies the body of Mary McPhie –
laid to rest by a JCB.

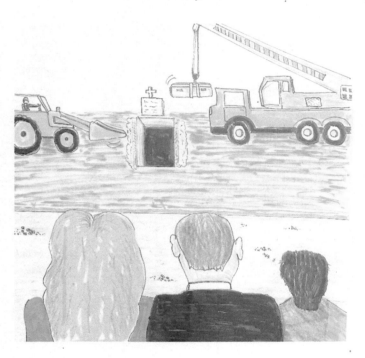

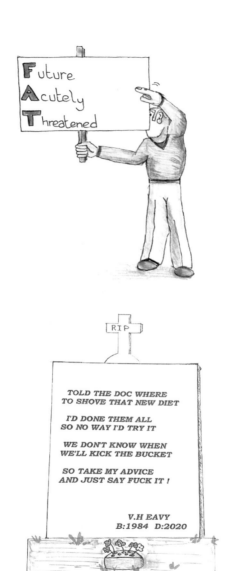

Another aspect of coming face-to-face with reality can be when booking holidays or even just public transport.

Many tour operators, and even mainstream airlines, carry advice for the obese traveller. Often this is based on 'health and safety' and relates to the increased risk of deep vein thrombosis (blood clots in the veins of the leg which can be dangerous) which is commoner in overweight air travellers. However, carrying excess baggage of all types involves extra cost and, on some airlines, morbidly obese travellers may have to buy an extra seat. One airline labels this as an 'extra comfort seat' but we know what they mean.

Things are moving in a similar direction for rail travel with high-speed travel on trains firmly on the horizon. One of the stipulations for companies bidding to provide high-speed rail travel in the UK is a provision of wider seats, essentially for bigger posteriors. Unfortunately, along with this is a plan for reduced numbers of steps up into the carriages. This suggests that those with physical challenges might be more comfortable when inside the train but experience difficulty actually boarding it in the first place.

The GOOD NEWS is that using public transport and just simply doing more walking reduces BMI.

The Doc and Mr Don't Know

Question: Which diet should I follow?

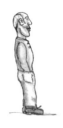

Mr Don't Know: Rather than follow someone else's diet with foodstuffs that you don't even like, why don't you devise your own? Name it after yourself and, when it works, all your pals and relatives will be clamouring for the details. A win-win for all involved.

Doc: Whichever diet you decide to follow remember to choose one that is realistic which can evolve into your maintenance or regular diet.

When people talk about surgery following weight loss it often relates to the removal of excess skin. A tummy tuck, which many people joke about, must hold the prize for being among the most mutilating of procedures leaving the patient with a scar from hip to hip.

This can be even worse for the ten percent of people who form keloid scars, which become thickened and raised.

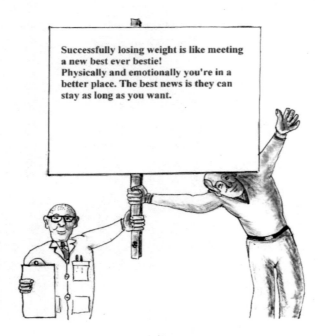

The Doc and Mr Don't Know

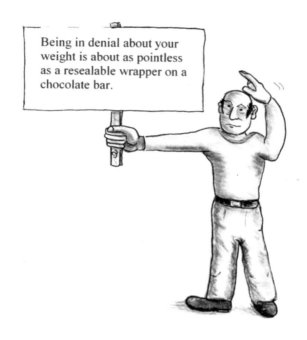

Being in denial about your weight is about as pointless as a resealable wrapper on a chocolate bar.

We all know that the number of people over their ideal weight has 'ballooned' but why should this have happened?

It's not as if the genetics of the entire population has changed. Neither can all overweight folks blame it on the hormones.

But we do know is that over the last 50 years, the food industry has gradually increased the number of calories we eat chiefly in the form of sugars. Back in the day, the thinking was carbohydrates (which breaks down into sugars) had less calories than fat and this in turn helped push the idea of low-fat diets.

Unfortunately, swiftly broken-down carbohydrates create a sugar 'high' which causes the body to produce insulin.

Insulin in turn lowers blood sugar by storing the energy from sugars as fat. The more sugars we consume, the more insulin we produce, which can result in us carrying more fat than we are able to use.

In these circumstances, our stomachs begin to fool us that we are still hungry even when we have had enough to eat by producing a hormone called Ghrelin.

In normal situations the greedy ghrelin is balanced by 'levelling leptins', another hormone group which make us feel full. But it is a continual imbalance between these hormones, driven by carbohydrates in the form of sugars, that is partly responsible for our weight gain.

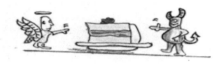

Leptin the Leveller vs Greedy Ghrelin

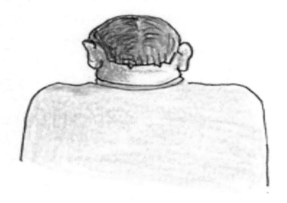

What's Causing My Fat Increase?

Now we need to look at the factors causing these imbalances. Some are bad habits, some lifestyle-related, some caused by disease and some as a result of situations we can only influence in modest ways.

Situations leading to weight gain include:

- Snacking
- Stress
- Depression
- Alcohol misuse
- Dieting

Snacking

People gain weight from snacking because they do not consider eating small meal amounts between main meals to count – it absolutely does!

Depression

Being depressed is a powerful cause of being overweight because a quick sugar rush from eating produces feel-good hormones, albeit only for a short period of time.

Unfortunately, if being overweight provokes anxiety then depression may get worse and the vicious spiral continues.

Dieting

Yes – believe it or not, dieting can cause weight gain! Although dieting increases Ghrelin levels, the balance between the greedy and the levelling hormones settles down as long as a sensible diet is followed. If dieting is interrupted by intermittent bingeing however, ultimately the bad guys win, since the body's reaction is to carry on trying to gain weight.

Alcohol

Alcohol in moderation, like most things, doesn't impact on weight very much. However, having six pints of beer or a bottle of wine with a meal doesn't so much complement it, as swamp it!

Lack of Sleep

Lack of sleep from whatever cause is associated with being overweight. Whether it's having more time to eat or more complex reasons, the tendency is to end up with more calories in and less calories out.

Feet Factoid

Obesity often leads to severe feet problems. The pressure of excess weight on the feet flattens them and can cause significant pain. This in turn makes exercise difficult. Shoe choice is affected too.

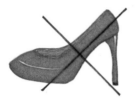 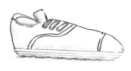

UK obesity rates have almost quadrupled in the last 25 years.

The Doc and Mr Don't Know

. **Mr Don't Know:** If those rates continue, is it possible the earth will be knocked off its axis?

Doc: No, but they are likely to destabilise the NHS budget..

The Doc and Mr Don't Know

Question: I'm considering a tummy tuck and would like to know a bit more about it. Do I have to pay for it and if so, how much does it cost?

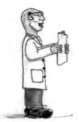

Doc: A tummy tuck, or abdominoplasty is surgery to improve the shape of the abdomen. It can involve removing excess loose skin, fat and stretch marks and tightening the abdomen. As it is regarded as aesthetic surgery, it is not usually available on the NHS. The average cost of abdominoplasty is between £4000 and £6000.

Mr Don't Know: One way of raising money to pay for the surgery could be by reducing your spend on non-essential foodstuffs.

By the time you've saved the money for the surgery, you may have lost enough weight and it's no longer needed… And you now have loads of extra money to spend!

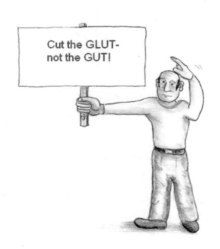

'A pill for every illness, an operation for everything else', may sound like an attractive idea but being overweight isn't a disease albeit it can result in an awful lot of them, so tablets don't necessarily work.

There is in fact one drug on the market which can be prescribed by GPs for obesity but to get any benefit from it you already have to be on a low-calorie diet.

And of course, nothing comes free. This drug is associated with a range of side effects from abdominal pain and diarrhoea to non-absorption of essential vitamins. Other drugs being trialled for obesity can have similar side effects.

An operation just to sort things out quickly may seem even more attractive but the truth is somewhat awkward.

'Bariatric surgery' for obesity is currently proving very popular and usually involves a keyhole surgery to squeeze bits of the gut so that we have the sensation of being full of food.

One of the commonest procedures is 'gastric banding' in which a silicone band is placed around the stomach to stop it filling too much. As the stomach is the first part of the gut to store food before it continues its downward journey, the stomach feels more full with a smaller meal. Whilst this operation can be effective, an operation still involves making decisions.

Way back when one of us was a cop on the beat, and the other had hair, the 'in' operation for obese people was jaw-wiring. This procedure sounded and looked like a horror movie scene where the victim, sorry, patient had his/her jaw wired to such an extent that it would only open wide enough to accept small volumes of food.

Rather unfortunately at around the same time (particularly for some denizens of Glasgow) food processors and food

109

mixers became widely available. With the right mix established, patients with wired jaws could consume large volumes of Mars bars through a straw!

Rather unbelievably, having opted for an operation to assist with weight loss, and with it better health prospects, they instead chose to circumvent it!

The same kinds of shenanigans are possible following operations such as gastric banding usually though, to get to the stage of needing that kind of operation you would have needed to demonstrate an ability to achieve substantial weight loss in the first place.

Paying for bariatric surgery either to make you feel full after a meal or stop you absorbing food, can be highly effective with very few people dying with possible complications. However, if you then choose to make smoothies out of chocolate bars, your money is wasted…and the weight just goes back on.

As an overweight person we go food shopping in a supermarket. Despite foodstuffs carrying calorific values in respect of fat, carbohydrates, sugar etc, we choose to ignore the labelling, buying and consuming without concern for the consequences. Piling on the pounds, we can all be guilty of then looking for someone/something to blame for our weight gain. But that's about the same as approaching a farmer's field with a sign on the gate, warning 'Bull in field', choosing to enter anyway, and immediately blaming the farmer when the bull charges!

So, whether we point the finger at the government, sugar manufacturers, poor labelling, or even Santa Claus for bringing us too many sweets, we really should try to stop this blame game.

Taking responsibility for our own actions is a bedrock principal in everything we do, including successful weight loss. It really comes back to what we said earlier:

We Really Have to Want to Lose Weight.

Successfully losing weight comes down to whether we value ourselves enough to believe we are worth it.

So if you are ready to commit, here's what we suggest:

Look at yourself in a mirror and envisage stepping out of your fat suit… Seeing yourself emerge as a new healthier happier individual. This is <u>absolutely</u> possible and does not have to be difficult.

Next decide the best way to do it for you. Our advice would be to choose the path of least resistance, the easiest way to lose weight and keep it off. Although some folk can find the commitment a bit daunting, remember the old adage:

The Longest Journey Begins with The First Step.

Sculptors and carvers often say that their work simply releases objet d'art already within the piece and it's exactly the same with our bodies. For most of us, the shape we'd love to be is just waiting to be released. With a few strategic cuts to our food intake, we can soon reveal that new shape.

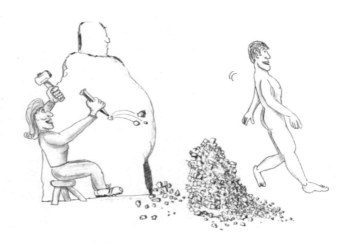

The way Kenny did it was to follow the 5/2 fast diet* by Dr Michael Mosley. In essence it involved eating less on two, non-consecutive days, of a seven-day period. It seemed brilliantly easy, and it was effective. Even if reverting to our excessive eating on the five non-diet days, the two days of reduced intake equates to a noticeable drop in calories consumed, meaning there is still progressive weight loss. It is also an easy method to dip back into if you find yourself falling off the wagon, as you're free to choose any two days in the week that suit you best. Essentially you can tailor your diet to suit your lifestyle. This is just one method but one that suited Kenny's lifestyle. Successfully losing weight is a bit like getting our teeth whitened – it's instantly and reassuringly noticeable, like the gift that keeps on giving!

Whichever way you choose, stick with it, and you too will become a fat loser... In the nicest way possible!

*As always check with your own doctor to ensure any weight loss path is suitable for you.

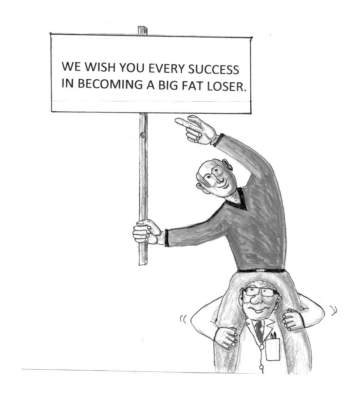

WHEN CONGRATULATING A FRIEND WHO'S SHED WEIGHT, BE CAREFUL HOW YOU PHRASE THEIR ACHIEVEMENT...

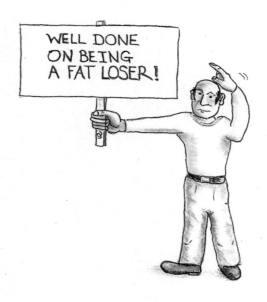